THE BIBLE CURE®

FOR

CANDIDA AND YEAST INFECTIONS

SILOAM

A STRANG COMPANY

THE BIBLE CURE FOR CANDIDA AND YEAST INFECTIONS
by Don Colbert, M.D.
Published by Siloam
A Strang Company
600 Rinehart Road
Lake Mary, Florida 32746
www.siloam.com

Unless otherwise noted, all Scripture quotations are from the Holy Bible, New Living Translation, copyright © 1996. Used by permission of Tyndale House Publishers, Inc., Wheaton, Illinois 60189.

Scripture quotations marked NKJV are from the New King James Version of the Bible. Copyright © 1979, 1980, 1982 by Thomas Nelson, Inc., publishers. Used by permission.

Scripture quotations marked NAS are from the New American Standard Bible. Copyright © 1960, 1962, 1963, 1968, 1971, 1972, 1973, 1975, 1977 by the Lockman Foundation. Used by permission. (www.Lockman.org)

Library of Congress Catalog Card Number: 00-112300
International Standard Book Number: 0-88419-743-3

This book is not intended to provide medical advice
or to take the place of medical advice and treatment
from your personal physician. Readers are advised to
consult their own doctors or other qualified health
professionals regarding the treatment of their medical problems. Neither the publisher nor the author
takes any responsibility for any possible conse-
quences from any treatment, action or application of
medicine, supplement, herb or preparation to any
person reading or following the information in this
book. If readers are taking prescription medications,
they should consult with their physicians and not
take themselves off of medicines to start supplemen-
tation without the proper supervision of a physician.

06 07 08 09 10 — 16 15 14 13 12
Printed in the United States of America

You Can
Reclaim Your Health

Perhaps you've picked up this book wondering just what a Bible cure is all about. Maybe you've never before considered that God genuinely cares for your health. This Bible verse explains how He feels about your sicknesses.

"Wherever he [Jesus] went, he healed people of every sort of disease and illness. He felt great pity for the crowds that came, because their problems were so great and they didn't know where to go for help. They were like sheep without a shepherd" (Matt. 9:35–36).

Not only does He care, but He also has great power to defeat all disease and sickness. God is greater than any disease or sickness that you will ever experience. The Bible says this about Jesus Christ: "Therefore also God highly exalted Him, and bestowed on Him the name which is above every name, that at the name of Jesus EVERY KNEE SHOULD BOW, of those who are in heaven, and on earth, and under the earth" (Phil. 2:9–10, NAS).

This verse simply says that Jesus Christ is higher and bigger than anything you will ever encounter. He is greater than all sickness and every disease. Because of that, every sickness and disease—no matter how great or small—must bow. That is the secret of His healing power.

You may have never before considered a Bible cure as an option in dealing with candida or yeast. If not, then get ready to reclaim your health in an entirely new way!

Candida, Candidiasis and Yeast Infections

Candida, candidiasis or the yeast syndrome is simply an overgrowth of yeast, usually in the intestinal tract and other tissues of the body. In women, painful yeast infections that infect the vagina can cause PMS and reduced sex drive.

Yeast can also overgrow in the GI tract, causing heartburn, indigestion, abdominal bloating, cramps, constipation or diarrhea, nausea and gas. Excessive yeast overgrowth is also related to environmental sensitivities and illnesses that heighten sensitivities to foods, chemicals such as smoke, chemical odors from carpets and fabrics and auto exhaust.

Yeast is everywhere. It's found in the food we eat and in the air we breathe, so it's impossible to avoid exposure to it. As a matter of fact, yeast normally lives in the human body. It flourishes in the warm, moist environment of the GI and vaginal tracts.

Still, you don't have to suffer from painful yeast attacks and overgrowth. There's a better way.

A Bold, New Approach

With the help of the practical and faith-inspiring wisdom contained in this Bible Cure booklet, combined with alternative healing methods, you can beat yeast infections naturally.

Through the power of good nutrition, healthy lifestyle choices, exercise, vitamins and supplements, and most importantly of all, through the power of dynamic faith, you can halt the painful symptoms of debilitating yeast imbalances.

Enduring the pain and discomfort of candida and yeast syndrome is not God's will for you. With God's grace, perfect health and increasing joy await you!

So, as you read this book, prepare to triumph in your battle against candidiasis and yeast syndrome. This Bible Cure booklet is filled with practical steps, hope, encouragement and valuable information on how to develop a healthy, empowered lifestyle. In this book, you will

*uncover God's divine plan of health
for body, soul and spirit
through modern medicine, good nutrition
and the medicinal power
of Scripture and prayer.*

You will also discover life-changing scriptures throughout this booklet that will strengthen and encourage you.

As you read, apply and trust God's promises, you will also uncover powerful Bible Cure prayers to help you line up your thoughts and feelings with God's plan of divine health for you—a plan that includes living victoriously. In this Bible Cure booklet, you will find powerful insight in the following chapters:

You can confidently take the natural and spiritual steps outlined in this book to defeat candidiasis and yeast syndrome forever.

It is my prayer that these practical suggestions for health, nutrition and fitness will bring whole-ness to your life—body, soul and spirit. May they deepen your fellowship with God and strengthen your ability to worship and serve Him.

—Don Colbert, M.D.

A Bible Cure Prayer
FOR YOU

Lord, You have revealed the causes for yeast syndrome, and in You are the reme-dies, cures and methods of prevention. Guide and direct me in applying this Bible cure method. Consecrate me, body, mind and spirit, to walk in divine health. Amen.

Chapter 1

Get Informed

Whether you realize it or not, becoming better informed is actually a godly principle. The Bible says, "For the LORD grants wisdom! From his mouth come knowledge and understanding. He grants a treasure of good sense to the godly" (Prov. 2:6–7).

Wouldn't you like for God to grant you a treasure of good sense regarding your health? Of course you would! Getting God's wisdom and good sense begins with becoming better informed. In this chapter we will take a good look at candidiasis and yeast infections and develop a better understanding of the various causes for this painful problem and what can be done naturally to cure it.

Candidiasis, a Closer Look

Yeast is actually a single-celled organism found everywhere: in water, air and on land. Candida is also present in all people from the first few months of life and usually lives harmoniously with us. What's destructive about yeast is how it can change from a harmless form to a dangerous invader.

When it changes forms, candida overgrowth can affect nearly every organ in the body and particularly the GI tract, nervous system, genital/urinary tract, endocrine system and immune system.

Under normal conditions yeast lives in our bodies without causing us any problems. Nearly three pounds of friendly bacteria in our intestines help to keep it in check. These friendly bacteria help our bodies maintain a balance of power between the good bacteria and the yeast.

That's until we upset this delicate balance with antibiotics, prednisone, hormones such as estrogen and progesterone, too much stress, diabetes or by eating too much sugar and highly processed foods. These things can swing the balance of power, causing an overgrowth of yeast to occur.

If this happens when your immune system is weakened, the harmless yeast can transform itself into an invasive fungal form.

This invasive form, called "mycelial form," actually produces root-like tentacles called "rhizoids." These roots can then penetrate through the lining of the GI tract, causing a painful condition known as "leaky gut," which is increased intestinal permeability. When you have a leaky gut, partially digested food particles are able to pass through the intestinal lining and directly enter the bloodstream. Not only that, but toxic waste produced by the candida passes right into the bloodstream, too. When this happens, food allergies can result, as well as symptoms of excessive bloating, gas, belching, heartburn, diarrhea and constipation.

> Then David asked the Lord, "Should I chase them? Will I catch them?" And the LORD told him, "Yes, go after them. You will surely recover everything that was taken from you!"
> —1 SAMUEL 30:8

What Are the Symptoms?

Yeast produces more than seventy-nine known toxins. But probably the worst toxic substance produced by yeast is acetaldehyde. When this substance enters into the liver, it is then converted into alcohol. Acetaldehyde contributes to a raft of harmful symptoms. Here are a few of them:

- Fatigue
- Mental cloudiness
- Disorientation
- Confusion
- Irritability
- Headaches
- Anxiety
- Depression

Not only does yeast produce these distressing symptoms, but it also depletes minerals, increases free radical formation and disrupts enzymes needed to produce energy.

So you can see that yeast can invade the body, wreaking havoc wherever it goes. It also produces many different toxins that can make you feel absolutely miserable.

If yeast is given enough time, it can invade the bloodstream and may affect any organ or tissue in the entire body. As soon as a particular organ in your body is affected, symptoms begin to occur. For instance, as candida or its toxic waste products affect the nervous system, you may begin to experience the following symptoms:

- Fatigue
- Memory loss
- Insomnia
- Depression
- Mood swings
- Sleepiness
- Attention-deficit disorder
- Hyperactivity
- Autistic tendencies

An Avalanche of Physical Complaints

Left unchecked, candida overgrowth can sweep through your entire body like an avalanche. Before long every organ system can be affected. If your body is under a yeast attack, you may feel extremely fatigued much of the time. That's because yeast will often affect the endocrine system, eventually causing adrenal exhaustion and chronic fatigue. Thyroid problems can also be related to yeast overgrowth, including both over-active and underactive thyroid function. Skin problems such as eczema, hives, psoriasis and acne can develop, too.

As your body struggles to fight off the ravages of yeast overgrowth, eventually your immune system can be compromised. Food allergies may begin to surface as well as other food sensitivities.

Once candida weakens the digestive system, it becomes increasingly difficult to break down proteins into amino acids. When the partially digested proteins, called peptides, are absorbed directly into the bloodstream, your immune system recognizes them as foreign invaders. At this point your body may begin to form antibodies to attack them.

Often this immune reaction takes place in the

lining of the small intestine, which therefore causes even more damage to the small intestines, leading to increased intestinal permeability, or leaky gut. A vicious cycle of destruction and allergic reactions spiral out of control.

Candida overgrowth in the small intestines can rob your body of vital nutrients. The toxic poisons that are excreted can poison your body's tissues.

What Causes Candida?

The most common reason that yeast grows out of control is due to excessive use of antibiotics. Many people have recurrent sinus infections, recurrent bladder infections, recurrent bouts of bronchitis or strep throat or prostatitis.

Many teenagers have severe acne and are on antibiotics such as tetracycline for years. Many times the acne is actually the result of candida. So, the acne may actually worsen rather than improve on tetracycline.

Because these people have repeatedly used antibiotics or have been on long-term antibiotics, these drugs eventually kill the majority of the good bacteria that live in the GI tract. Since the antibiotics do not affect candida, they multiply rapidly and may proliferate out of control. The yeast are normally held in check by the friendly bacteria, which have been killed by the antibiotics.

Antibiotics and Our Meat Supply

In addition, people who eat large amounts of beef, pork, chicken and veal will usually absorb small amounts of antibiotics and hormone residues. In 1991, the Centers for Disease Control in Atlanta revealed that half of the fifteen million pounds of antibiotics produced in America each year are used on livestock and poultry.[1] Many of the cattle, pigs and poultry have antibiotics added to their food routinely. As a result, residues of these antibiotics remain in many of the meats we eat.

Long-term antibiotics taken for chronic infections or consumed by eating large amounts of meat will eventually affect the delicate balance of good bacteria in the GI tract, leading to death of the good bacteria and an overgrowth of yeast.

Also, successive use of antibiotics is causing the development of resistant strains of bacteria. Antibiotic resistance is much more common when antibiotics are used frequently. If this trend continues, many infectious diseases may be almost impossible to treat due to antibiotic resistance.

Side Effects From the Pill

Birth control pills and the hormone proges-terone are factors in developing candida over-growth. When progesterone levels are high, such as during the second half of the menstrual cycle or during pregnancy, women are much more prone to develop yeast vaginitis. Corticosteroids such as prednisone are commonly associated with yeast overgrowth.

Do You Have Candida?

We know that everyone has candida. Yes, it is actually present in all our GI tracts. But is the yeast in your body in balance with the good bac-teria? Or is it growing out of control? This is extremely difficult to assess. Even lab test results are often unclear about it, even in very severe states of overgrowth.

Most medical doctors do not recognize can-dida as a problem in normal people. However, they recognize thrush in an AIDS victim and treat it immediately. But since most people's immune systems never become so compromised, the kind of extreme overgrowth of yeast seen in an AIDS patient is rarely seen in the normal population.

Nevertheless, even when candida overgrowth is not life-threatening, still it is able to produce the symptoms recognized as candidiasis or the yeast syndrome.

> *He had heard that Hezekiah had been very sick and that he had recovered.*
> —Isaiah 39:1

Most nutritional doctors will diagnose candidiasis based on a detailed medical history and a yeast questionnaire. Occasionally he or she will request that a comprehensive digestive stool analysis be taken. This careful examination of the stool helps your doctor to evaluate how well your food is being digested and absorbed, to check for parasites, to identify the presence of beneficial and pathogenic bacteria and to identify excessive yeast overgrowth.

I routinely have my patients complete the yeast questionnaire developed by Dr. William Crook.[2]

A BIBLE CURE HEALTH TIP

What About You?

Would you like to know if your own health problems are yeast-related? Then answer the questions below and add up your points to see how you stack up.[3]

1. Have you taken tetracycline or other antibiotics for acne for one month or longer? 25

2. Have you ever taken other broad-spectrum antibiotics for respiratory, urinary or other infections for two months or longer, or in short courses four or more times in one year? 20

3. Have you ever taken a broad-spectrum antibiotic (even a single course)? 6

4. Have you ever been bothered by persistent prostatitis, vaginitis or other problems affecting your reproductive organs? 25

5. Have you been pregnant . . .
   One time? 3
   Two or more times? 5

6. Have you taken birth control pills . . .
   For six months to two years? 8
   For more than two years? 15

7. Have you taken prednisone or other cortisone-type drugs . . .
   For two weeks or less? 6
   For more than two weeks? 15

8. Does exposure to perfumes, insecticides, fabric shop odors and other chemicals provoke . . .
   Mild symptoms? 5
   Moderate to severe symptoms? 20

9. Are your symptoms worse on damp, muggy days or in moldy places? 20

10. Have you had athlete's foot, ringworm, "jock-itch" or other chronic infections of the skin or nails?
   Mild to moderate? .10
   Severe or persistent? 20

11. Do you crave sugar? 10

12. Do you crave breads? .10

13. Do you crave alcoholic beverages? 10

14. Does tobacco smoke really bother you? 10

If you are a woman and scored over 180, or a man and scored over 140, yeast-connected problems are almost certainly present.

If you are a woman and scored 120–180, or a man and scored 90–140, yeast-connected health problems are probably present.

If you are a woman and scored 60–119, or a man and scored 40–89, yeast-connected health problems are possibly present.

If you are a woman and scored less than 60, or a man and scored less than 40, yeast-connected health problems are less likely present.

Knowing the Score

So, how did you score? Knowing where you

stand is essential in your battle against yeast syndrome. Whether you scored higher or lower than you expected really doesn't matter. By reading this booklet, you hold in your hands valuable keys to overcoming the distressing yeast syndrome forever. Let's take a look at your body's main defense team against candida: your incredible immune system.

Your Incredible Defense Team

It's vital for you to improve immune function to overcome the yeast syndrome. The immune system is how your body protects itself against yeast, fungi, bacteria, viruses, cancer cells and other foreign invaders. Chances are that if you have chronic candida, then you may also have a depressed immune system.

If the cells of your immune system formed a football team, the white blood cells would play defense. White blood cells are actually produced in the bone marrow, but they are found in large numbers in the blood and in lymphoid tissues. The lymphoid tissues include the thymus, spleen and lymph nodes.

The thymus gland is the quarterback—it's a main player in the immune system's defense against yeast. That's why strengthening your thymus can help you win against candida.

The thymus is a small gland located under the upper breastbone, which produces helper T-cells that rally other white blood cells into action. When a helper T-cell recognizes that an invader like yeast is attacking the body, it signals to B-cells to make antibodies that are specific for that particular foreign invader. Antibodies then destroy the invader.

Other T-cells that are produced by the thymus include suppressor T-cells, which help to keep the B-cells in check. This

> *Lord,*
> *your discipline is*
> *good, for it leads to*
> *life and health.*
> —Isaiah 38:16

prevents them from overproducing antibodies. Natural killer cells are also stimulated by helper T-cells to kill tumor cells.

You can see how important the thymus gland is. When the thymus is weak, not only can yeast overgrow, but your body also becomes more susceptible to viral and bacterial infections. You also become more susceptible to cancer. The thymus is also important in protecting your body from autoimmune diseases like rheumatoid arthritis and lupus.

Building up your immune system is a powerful

and natural way to help your body score a winning touchdown against the yeast syndrome. In the following chapters we'll address some powerful ways to fortify your immune system's strength and help to free you from candida forever!

Conclusion

Yeast syndrome is not a chronic battle that you cannot win. It's not a life sentence of pain, distress and embarrassment. God is granting a treasure of wisdom and good sense to you about the yeast syndrome so that you can understand how it works and how you can work with your body to defeat it.

Wisdom, however, is just the first key. In the following chapters we will explore powerful ways you can strike back at the root of candida and destroy its hold on your body forever. By following the spiritual and natural keys presented within the following pages, you can restore your body's natural balance and reclaim your health.

A BIBLE CURE PRAYER
FOR YOU

Dear God, I thank You for the wisdom You are providing for me as the first key to becoming free of the yeast syndrome forever. I acknowledge that nothing is greater than You—You are higher and greater than all that concerns me physically, mentally and spiritually. I believe that You truly and genuinely care about all of my health concerns, and I thank You for Your great compassion. In Jesus' name, amen.

15

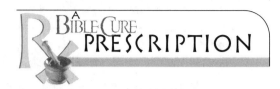

R A BIBLE CURE PRESCRIPTION

Did you take the yeast syndrome test in this chapter? If so, what was your score?

_____

What symptoms of yeast do you have on a chronic basis?

_____
_____
_____
_____
_____
_____
_____

Do you believe that God genuinely cares about everything about you—including all of your health issues?

_____
_____
_____
_____
_____

Chapter 2

Restore Your Health With Nutrition

You have already seen that the yeast syndrome can sweep through your body like a plague, robbing your energy and ravaging your health. But God is a restorer, and He promises to restore you back to health and vigor. The Bible says, "For I will restore you to health" (Jer. 30:17, NAS).

God does indeed promise full restoration. Again, the Bible says, "Then I will make up to you for the years that the swarming locust has eaten, the creeping locust, the stripping locust, and the gnawing locust" (Joel 2:25, NAS).

Let's look at a powerful Bible cure key to your total restoration and recovery: nutrition.

Dietary Factors You Should Know

In order to experience recovery from yeast overgrowth, it's critically important to make some

17

changes to your diet. Certain dietary factors promote candida overgrowth that you can control.

You will need to adhere strictly to a special diet for a period of time in order to experience full restoration of your body's natural balance. How long will depend upon the severity of your yeast syndrome, as candida ranges from extremely mild to very severe.

The majority of patients suffering from candida will need to stay on the diet for three months. Patients with severe candidiasis will need to stay on the diet six months to one year, and patients with mild candida may need to stay on the diet only one to two months.

> *He fills my life with good things. My youth is renewed like the eagle's.*
> —PSALM 103:5

Let's take a look at some dietary factors that promote yeast overgrowth.

Your Sweet Tooth

If you have a sweet tooth, you may have to wait to satisfy it. Believe it or not, the average American takes in about 150 pounds of sugar per person per year! Sugar-rich foods are the single most important contributing factor to candida overgrowth. That's why sugar must be strictly avoided for a season of time so that your body has a chance to reclaim its natural balance.

What you eat will determine how well your immune system is able to function. A high-sugar diet will impair immunity. This means all sugars, including the following:

- White sugar
- Brown sugar
- Syrups
- Honey
- Fructose
- Glucose
- Maltose
- Maple sugar
- Molasses
- Date sugar

Even the sugars found in fruit juices and high-sugar vegetable juices like carrot juice must be omitted. Fruits should be omitted for the first three weeks of the yeast-free diet. The herbal sweetener Stevia is an excellent alternative to sugar. Also, the new sugar substitute Splenda is acceptable in moderation.

Milk Products and You

Milk and milk products contain lactose, which also encourages candida growth. Small amounts of butter are acceptable for most individuals with less-severe cases of candida.

Lactose-free yogurt and kefir are exceptions.

They are actually good for you, for they contain good bacteria that help to restore bacteria in the bowel. Some people always make it a point to eat yogurt when taking antibiotics and certain other drugs that we will discuss later on. This can be especially helpful before yeast grows out of control. However, avoid kefir and yogurt that contain sugar, fruit or lactose, since these products will feed the yeast.

So, What About Fruit?

Fruit should be avoided for the first three weeks. After that you may reintroduce the less sweet fruits. Eat fruit by itself thirty minutes before your meals. Here's a list of fruit you can reintroduce into your diet:

- Lemons
- Limes
- Apples
- Kiwi
- Blackberries
- Grapefruits
- Watermelon
- Raspberries
- Strawberries
- Blueberries

Here are some sweet fruits to avoid:

- Dried fruits
- Bananas
- Cherries
- Oranges
- Cantaloupe
- Honeydew

- Grapes
- Peaches
- Plums
- Mangoes
- Pineapple

Dealing With Carbs

Most of us love carbs, especially when it comes to breads and snack foods. Nevertheless, while you are working with your body to restore it to natural balance, closely watching what carbohydrates you eat is vitally important.

Candida loves refined carbohydrates and thrives on them, so they actually become food for the candida rather than for you. By decreasing these refined carbohydrates, you will slow down the rate of multiplication of yeast cells. Here's a list of refined carbs to avoid:

- White bread
- Pasta
- Muffins
- Pancakes
- Most breakfast cereals
- Potato chips
- Corn chips
- White crackers

In addition to these food items, you will need to decrease your consumption of both packaged and processed foods. Most of these foods are highly processed. Refined sugar is added to this list as well. These foods are a perfect source to help yeast to multiply. Sugar and highly processed foods depress the immune system. All of these foods also have a high glycemic index. The glycemic index of a food is simply how rapidly a food causes the blood sugar to rise.[1]

Carbs You Can Choose

Some less-refined carbohydrates are actually good for you and highly desirable. As long as the following foods have not been refined, they are safe for you.

- Oats
- Millet bread
- Brown rice
- Spelt pasta
- Buckwheat
- Quinoa
- Amaranth
- Spelt

What About Whole Wheat?

If you have mild candida overgrowth, whole wheat may be fine for your diet. However, if your candida score fell into the moderate to severe range, then wheat is probably off limits for you, and you may be unable to tolerate whole wheat. If after eating whole-wheat products you develop bloating, belching, gas, drowsiness, irritability, mood changes or other symptoms of candida, you should avoid all wheat products for at least three months. Also, most whole-wheat products such as bread are made with yeast and therefore should be avoided.

Wheat is high in the protein gluten, and many individuals with candida overgrowth are gluten-sensitive. For such individuals, eating whole-wheat products may worsen their candida.

Therefore, if symptoms of candida occur after eating wheat products, stop eating grains for three months, and then reintroduce them slowly back into your diet, combining them primarily with vegetables.

Oats also contain gluten, but in lower amounts than wheat. Oats may need to be avoided if symptoms occur.

Other Foods to Avoid

Foods with yeast and mold

Avoid foods with high amounts of yeast or mold in them. These include all cheeses and most breads, pastries and other baked goods containing yeast. Yeast- or mold-containing foods do not make candida grow; however, they cause symptoms such as bloating, gas, belching, irritability and other symptoms because many are allergic or sensitive to yeast products.

Some condiments

Avoid condiments and sauces that contain yeast

such as mustard, ketchup, barbecue sauce, soy sauce, steak sauce and Worcestershire sauce. Other condiments high in yeast include pickles, sauerkraut, horseradish, relishes, miso, tempeh and tamari.

If you have mild symptoms of candida, these foods should be avoided for one to two months. Most patients should avoid them for three months. If you have severe symptoms of candida, you should avoid them six months to a year.

Vinegary foods

Foods containing vinegar should also be avoided. These include nearly all salad dressings, mayonnaise and mayonnaise products. Raw, unfiltered apple cider vinegar is one exception, however. If a patient with yeast has no symptoms of candida (such as bloating, belching, gas, irritability or mood changes), he may tolerate this very well because apple cider vinegar actually contains good bacteria that fight yeast proliferation. However, some patients with candida overgrowth cannot take any forms of vinegar.

Preserved and processed meats

Some specially prepared and preserved meats can be high in yeast. They include pickled and smoked meats and fish, sausages, corned beef, hot dogs, bacon, ham and pastrami.

Nuts

Nuts are often high in mold, especially when they are not stored in airtight containers in the refrigerator or freezer. To prevent nuts and seeds from getting moldy, purchase them in their shells and crack and eat them as you desire. However, avoid peanuts and cashews since they usually have a higher mold content. Patients with candida are usually allergic or sensitive to mold.

Mushrooms

Mold, as well as yeast foods, causes symptoms when a person is allergic or sensitive to yeast products. Avoid all types of mushrooms since these are fungi, and yeast is simply a form of fungus.

Leftovers

Discard all leftovers after a day or two since they tend to grow mold.

Alcoholic beverages

Alcoholic beverages (such as beer) contain a high content of yeast and should be avoided.

Allergy-causing foods

Finally, the last group of foods that you must avoid is allergy-causing foods. Commonly, food allergies involve the following foods:

- Eggs
- Dairy products
- Wheat
- Corn
- Yeast
- Chocolate
- Citrus fruits

To determine if you have food allergies or sensitivities, you can have a RAST test. For more information on food allergies, read my booklet *The Bible Cure for Allergies*.

What Can I Eat?

Now that we have talked about all the foods that you should avoid, let's talk about all the foods that you can eat. Vegetables are one of the most important foods for a person with candida overgrowth. You should eat a minimum of three to five servings of vegetables a day.

Virtuous Vegetables

Even though it's best to eat vegetables raw, you can lightly steam or stir-fry them as well. You can also make many varieties of delicious vegetable soup.

If you have candida, just avoid these veggies: potatoes, mushrooms and sweet potatoes. Potatoes and sweet potatoes have a high glycemic index, which feeds yeast. Mushrooms are a yeast food.

Eat at least three to five servings of the following vegetables a day (a serving equals either 1 cup cooked or 2 cups raw):

- Artichokes
- Avocados
- Green beans
- Broccoli
- Cabbage
- Cauliflower
- Chard
- Cucumbers
- Garlic
- Lettuce (all types)
- Onions
- Parsnips
- Green bell peppers
- Radishes
- Soybeans
- Sprouts
- Squash (yellow, summer)
- Water chestnuts
- Asparagus
- Beans
- Beet greens
- Brussels sprouts
- Carrots
- Celery
- Eggplant
- Greens (kale, chard, mustard, collard, spinach turnip)
- Parsley
- Peppers
- Hot chili peppers
- Snow peas
- Spinach
- Alfalfa sprouts
- Tomatoes
- Turnips
- Zucchini

(You can make a delicious soup with a combination of these vegetables.)

Beans or legumes are high in protein and have about the same amount of calories as grains. They are also very high in fiber and include black beans, black-eyed peas, garbanzo beans, kidney beans, lentils, lima beans, pinto beans, red beans, soybeans and split peas. When legumes are combined with grains, they form a complete protein.

Powerful Proteins

Meats, poultry and fish do not feed candida. However, some animals are fed antibiotics, which remain in meat and can cause yeast to proliferate. That's why it is important for you to choose meat and poultry that are free of antibiotics, such as free-range beef and chicken.

Try to eat fish at least three times a week. Choose fatty fish such as salmon, herring, mackerel, halibut or sardines since they have a high content of Omega-3 fatty acids. You may also have lamb or veal.

Eggsxactly!

Finally, you may eat two to three servings of eggs each week, unless you are allergic to them. Just be sure to cook them well.

Fabulous Fats

The right fats add zest to your meals, and they are very healthy for your body. The fabulous fats allowed on the diet include extra-virgin olive oil, flaxseed oil, organic butter and cold-pressed vegetable oil such as safflower oil.

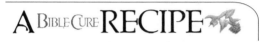

A BIBLE CURE RECIPE

REALLY GOOD SALAD DRESSING

Some of my patients have complained that they cannot eat salads on this diet because it contains vinegar. Well, here's a salad dressing you can make that is really good!

2 Tbsp. extra-virgin olive oil
1 Tbsp. freshly squeezed lemon juice
(or apple cider vinegar if you have no symptoms with it)
1 Tbsp. purified water
1 tsp. tarragon
1 tsp. garlic salt
1 tsp. parsley flakes
Dash of pepper
Dash of salt
2–3 drops Stevia (sweeten to taste)

Shake in cruet or jar. Pour over salad.

Meal Planning for the Candida Diet

Here are some helpful meal suggestions to get you started on your candida diet.

Breakfast

Day 1

- Egg omelet with sliced onion, tomatoes and peppers
- 1 slice millet, spelt or yeast-free rye toast or rice toast
- 1 pat organic butter

Day 2

- Old-fashioned oatmeal with cinnamon and almonds (cooked in water instead of milk)
- Sweeten with Stevia or Splenda
- 1 pat organic butter

Day 3

- Toasted rice or millet bread
- Top with almond butter spread

Day 4

- 2 scrambled eggs
- Toasted millet bread
- Brown rice
- 1 pat organic butter

Day 5
- Sunflower and sesame seeds mixed with hot oat bran cereal

Day 6
- Oat, rice, spelt or amaranth pancakes
- Raspberries, blackberries, strawberries or blueberries
- Sprinkle with Stevia or Splenda (This one must be eaten three weeks after the beginning of the candida program since fruits are introduced at this time.)

Day 7
- Organic plain low-fat yogurt or kefir with 1 tsp. acidophilus powder
- Fresh berries
- Sweeten with Stevia or Splenda (Again, this should be added three weeks after the beginning of the program. Also, realize that some people may not tolerate fruit with pancakes, so they may need to eat it thirty minutes before eating the pancakes or the yogurt.)

Lunches or Dinners

Day 1
- Baked, broiled or grilled chicken
- Brown rice
- Lima beans

Day 2
- Broiled, baked or grilled fish
- Green beans
- Broccoli

Day 3
- Turkey
- Lima beans
- Asparagus
- 1 slice millet bread
- 1 pat organic butter

Day 4
- 4 oz. free-range, lean filet mignon
- Brown rice
- Asparagus

Day 5
- Tuna fish sandwich
- Millet bread
- Lettuce, tomato and onions

Day 6
- Cornish hen
- Black-eyed peas
- Cooked carrots

Day 7
- Grilled salmon
- Green peas
- Broccoli

Feel free to add a salad to any one of these dinners. In addition, add all the vegetables you want. Just avoid croutons, cheese and most dressings. You may use the salad dressing recipe on page 29. Also, you may eat vegetable soup with any vegetables that are listed.

So, How Long?

If you have candida, expect to go on this program for one to six months, depending upon the severity of your symptoms. If your symptoms are severe, maintain the program for six months. If moderate, go on the program for three months. If your symptoms are mild, one to two months will be all the time you need. Go off the program when you have been symptom free at least one to three months.

Eating to Improve Your Immune System

Even after you've completed the candida diet regimen and your yeast is under control, you will still want to continue to strengthen your immune system through ongoing good nutrition. A strong immune system will overcome yeast attacks and protect your body from future invasions.

A diet high in saturated fat, such as animal fats, butter, cheese and whole milk, impairs immune function. But whole natural foods such as vegetables, fruits, whole grains, beans, seeds and nuts will help to improve the immune system. Also, Omega-3 fatty acids, such as what is found in fatty fish such as salmon and mackerel, strengthens the immune system. Flaxseed oil, evening primrose oil and black currant oil all help to improve the immune system as well.

Eating enough protein helps your immune system by increasing the production of antibodies that fight off bacteria and other invaders. And be sure to drink plenty of clean, filtered water—at least two quarts every day. But avoid chlorinated tap water that destroys friendly bacteria and can cause an overgrowth of yeast.

A Word About Food Allergies

If you scored high on the test for yeast syndrome, I encourage you to get tested for food allergies and sensitivities since they can play an integral role in the development of yeast syndrome.

Many individuals have food allergies and food sensitivities. You could be one of them. It's critically important to identify, eliminate or desensitize food allergies to properly restore immune function. Food allergies cause food that should be nourishing our bodies to create allergic reactions in our GI tracts.

What's Leaky Gut?

Food allergies are often related to a problem called "leaky gut." Leaky gut occurs when the lining of our intestines, which is supposed to absorb food and act as a barrier to keep out invading organisms, lies down on the job. This can happen when candida damages our GI tract.

Leaky gut opens a door for bacteria, yeast, viruses, parasites and undigested food molecules, as well as yeast and their toxic waste products, to enter the bloodstream. They then begin circulating. The partially digested food molecules activate the immune system, creating food allergies and food sensitivities. This further damages the lining of the GI tract, creating symptoms of fatigue, rashes, diarrhea, abdominal pain, memory loss, arthritis, autoimmune diseases, psoriasis and acne.

> *But those who wait on the LORD will find new strength. They will fly high on wings like eagles. They will run and not grow weary. They will walk and not faint.*
> —ISAIAH 40:31

When yeast overgrowth damages the intestinal

walls, it becomes difficult for friendly bacteria to recolonize the area. Pretty soon large molecules of incompletely digested food protein and yeast by-products begin to enter into the bloodstream, provoking immune responses. This in turn creates food allergies or sensitivities to numerous commonly eaten foods. It also causes food allergies or sensitivities to practically all yeast products such as mushrooms, soy sauce and breads with yeast.

You can see that a leaky gut creates a viscious cycle. When you eat a food that you're allergic or sensitive to, or when you eat a yeast-type food, the GI tract becomes inflamed and damages—and even destroys—cells in the intestines due to allergic reactions occurring in the lining of the intestines. As this process continues, it damages the intestinal tract even further and creates symptoms of bloating, gas, discomfort, diarrhea, spastic colon and nausea.

To rid your intestinal tract of yeast you must strengthen your immune system, repair the damaged intestinal tract, avoid foods that feed yeast or that you are allergic to, kill the yeast overgrowth with herbs and medication that we will look at later, repopulate the GI tract with good bacteria and at the same time sweep the excessive yeast overgrowth out with high-fiber foods.

Clearing up food allergies is extremely important in overcoming candida. I discuss this in detail in *The Bible Cure for Allergies*.

Fiber Facts

When you have a buildup of yeast and bacteria in your body, detoxifying is essential to restore you back to health.

One of the most important means of detoxifying the body is to have regular bowel movements on a daily basis, which means you must eat plenty of fiber and drink plenty of water.

You need at least 25–35 grams of fiber every day. The fiber intake of most Americans is far below this number. When you are dealing with an overgrowth of yeast, fiber helps to eliminate yeast so that it is not reabsorbed back into the body.

During the first week of your candida program, candida die-off reactions usually occur. When a yeast cell dies, it becomes food for another yeast cell, which tends to encourage the yeast colonies that are still present. The internal fluids of the dead yeast cells are feeding these yeast colonies. Therefore, it is critically important to eliminate these dead yeast cells through adequate fiber intake.

What You Need to Know About Fiber

Two types of fiber are available to you: soluble and insoluble fiber.

Soluble fiber

Examples of soluble fiber are listed as follows:

- Psyllium seed
- Fruit pectin
- Oat bran
- Rice bran

Soluble fiber actually feeds the good bacteria that live in the intestines. It ferments to produce short-chain fatty acids. These fatty acids nourish the cells in the large intestines, thus stimulating healing.

You need to get adequate amounts of soluble fiber, but not too much. Too much soluble fiber causes an overgrowth of intestinal bacteria, which in turn can create more problems for you by increasing bacterial toxins.

Insoluble fiber

Insoluble fiber is found in wheat bran and methylcellulose, which is a tasteless powder that gets swollen and gummy when wet. However, I don't recommend wheat bran for individuals with yeast overgrowth since many are sensitive to wheat products. Methylcellulose inactivates many toxins in the GI tract. It also stops bad bacteria and parasites from attacking the intestines, and it protects a person from developing increased gut permeability, which is worsening of the leaky gut.

To win your battle against candida you will need to eat high-fiber foods and take fiber supplements. A good fiber supplement is Ultrafiber by Metagenics, which contains barley bran, rice bran, cellulose, apple fiber, beet fiber and apple pectin. Take two scoops at bedtime with 8 ounces of water. You may also take two scoops upon awakening with a chlorophyll drink, which will be discussed later.

Improving Digestion

Not only are the foods you eat important in your battle against candida, but the way you eat your foods is just as important. Let's take a look at some ways you can assist your body by improving digestion.

- Drink a beverage about thirty minutes before eating.

- Digestion actually starts in the mouth, so it's critically important to mix the food you're eating with saliva. Your saliva contains enzymes that help to digest starches.

- Chew food slowly and thoroughly to break down the food properly. When it finally reaches the small intestines, it will be further broken down and assimilated more easily into the body.

- Take special care to chew meats and other protein foods extra thoroughly so that they can be digested properly in the stomach.

- Take one or two digestive enzymes with each meal. You may also take a hydrochloric acid supplement, one to two with each meal as recommended by your nutritionist. These may be purchased at a health food store. If you have a history of ulcer disease, gastritis or burning abdominal pains, consult your nutritional doctor prior to taking either of these supplements.

Believe it or not, if you have candida overgrowth and poor digestion, your body may be using most of your energy to digest your food. That's why you often feel exhausted.

What to Eat With What

Food combining has a powerful effect on digestion also. Food combining is especially important for candida sufferers. Here are some important food combining tips:

- Meats and proteins should not be eaten together with high-starch foods.

- Meats and proteins can be eaten with low-starch vegetables such as green beans, broccoli, cauliflower, asparagus and salads.

- Low-starch vegetables can also be eaten together with starchy vegetables such as potatoes and whole grains.

- Fruits should be eaten approximately thirty minutes before a meal and should be eaten alone.

Conclusion

Even if yeast has swept through your system like a plague of hungry locusts, stripping your intestines, gnawing away at your intestinal walls and breaking down your health by creeping into every organ system in your body, you are being armed with important and valuable weapons to defeat it. By giving you these vital keys, God has already begun to bring you full restoration. Believe God when He promises to restore to you the years that the plague of locusts has eaten. (See Joel 2:25.) God's promises are sure. He will not fail you!

A Bible Cure Prayer
FOR YOU

Dear God, thank You for beginning the process of total restoration for my body. Even though the yeast syndrome has attacked my body, Your power and wisdom are greater than every attack and every disease. Give me special divinely ordained grace to undergo a time of special dieting for candida. And help me to develop lifestyle changes that will set me free from the yeast syndrome attacks for the rest of my days. In Jesus' name, amen.

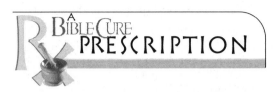

This diet is for the initial phase of your program and will be the strictest during this time. Candida feeds on certain foods, and these foods will need to be eliminated for a season.

Check the foods you will stop eating until your body's balance is restored.

- ❏ No sugar of any kind—white sugar, brown sugar, honey, molasses, barley, malt, rice syrup, etc.
- ❏ No artificial sweeteners—Sweet 'N Low, Nutra-Sweet, Equal, etc. (Stevia is allowed.)
- ❏ No fruit juice of any kind for the first three months, then gradually added back into diet if tolerated.
- ❏ No fruit of any kind for the first three weeks, then gradually added back into diet starting with low-glycemic fruits such as apples, kiwi, berries, grapefruit, lemons and limes.
- ❏ No dairy food of any kind—milk, cheese, cottage cheese, ice cream, sour cream, etc. (A small amount of organic butter, and yogurt and kefir with no lactose, sugar or fruit are acceptable.)
- ❏ No gluten grains of any kind found in wheat, rye, white or pumpernickel breads, or found

in pastry, crackers, etc. (Rice bread found in the frozen section of the health food store is a good replacement. Millet bread is also acceptable.) Oats contain less gluten, however, and may not be tolerated by those with severe candida.

❑ No foods containing yeast
❑ No breads or other bakery products containing yeast
❑ No alcoholic beverages of any kind
❑ No commercially prepared foods containing yeast
❑ No dry roasted nuts (Nuts in the shell—other than peanuts or cashews—are acceptable. The shell protects them from molding.)
❑ No vinegar and vinegar-containing foods with the possible exception of raw, unfiltered apple cider vinegar in those with mild candida.
❑ No soy sauce, tamari or natural root beer.
❑ No vitamin and mineral supplements containing yeast
❑ No pickled foods or smoked, dried or cured meats, including bacon
❑ No deep-fried foods of any kind
❑ No mushrooms

Chapter 3

Renew Your
Body With Supplements

Even if your body feels completely depleted by candida attack, God promises to renew your health and strength. The Bible says, "Bless the LORD, O my soul, and forget not all His benefits: Who forgives all your iniquities, who heals all your diseases, who redeems your life from destruction, who crowns you with lovingkindness and tender mercies, who satisfies your mouth with good things, so that your youth is renewed like the eagle's" (Ps. 103:2–5, NKJV).

Renewal comes from God. The Word of God declares, "But those who wait on the LORD shall renew their strength; they shall mount up with wings as eagles, they shall run and not be weary, and they shall walk and not faint" (Isa. 40:31, NKJV).

Renewal comes from God, but often He uses

natural methods to bring health and healing to you. He has filled the earth with many natural substances that, used with God's wisdom, can become instruments of His healing touch. For whether healing comes supernaturally or naturally, all healing comes from God, and all restoration is the benefit of His blessing.

Let's take a look at some of the powerful, natural herbs and other supplements for the third dynamic key of this Bible cure.

Supplements, Herbs and Medications

A number of natural herbs and supplements are powerfully effective against candida. In addition to your special candida diet, begin supplementing with sources of good bacteria. The lining of your GI tract has been a war zone and will need special healing, and any parasitic infestations you may have must also be addressed.

Let's look at some supplements that can help.

Garlic

One of the most important supplements for controlling yeast overgrowth is garlic. Allicin, the active ingredient in garlic, has powerful anti-fungal activity.

Take 500 milligrams of garlic three times a day.

Goldenseal

Goldenseal is included in the same family with Oregon grape and barberry. They are all in the berberines family. These potent natural substances contain extremely effective antifungal agents. These special agents actually activate macrophages, which are a type of white blood cell.

Berberines help to clear out bacterial over-growth in the small intestines, which commonly accompanies yeast overgrowth. Berberines also halt the bacterial and yeast enzymes that aggravate leaky gut. Many patients with chronic candidiasis have diarrhea. Berberines are also able to control diarrhea in many cases.

Take 500 milligrams of goldenseal three times a day for at least a month.

Grapefruit seed extract

Grapefruit seed extract, otherwise known as citrus extract, is a great supplement. It effectively kills both the candida and the parasite giardia, which may be associated with candida in some cases. However, it usually takes several months to eliminate the parasites.

Take 100–200 milligrams of grapefruit seed extract three times a day.

Caprylic acid

Caprylic acid is a long-chain fatty acid found in coconuts. It's extremely toxic to yeast, yet safe for humans. To be effective it must be taken in a time-released capsule.

Take 1000 milligrams of a time-released preparation with each meal.

Oil of oregano

Oil of oregano is a very good antifungal agent. It's more than one hundred times more potent than caprylic acid. I recommend oregano oil tablets from the nutritional company Biotics.

Take three 50-milligram tablets of oregano three times a day.

Tanalbit

Tanalbit is a plant extract that destroys yeast, including the spores, without harming good bacteria. It also contains natural tannins, which have intestinal antiseptic properties.

Take three capsules three times a day with each meal.

Chlorophyll supplements (green food)

Chlorophyll supplements, otherwise known as green food supplements, detoxify the colon and pack a powerful punch against candida. They boost the immune system as well. Chlorophyll keeps yeast and bacteria from spreading, and it even encourages the growth of friendly bacteria.

High-chlorophyll foods include wheat grass, barley grass, alfalfa, chlorella, spiralina and blue/green algae. All of these are obtained in Divine Health Green Superfood. (This is a supplement that I produce. It can be purchased by contacting my office or through the Internet at www.drcolbert.com.) These high-chlorophyll foods are very nutrient-dense and are excellent sources of essential amino acids, vitamins, minerals, essential fatty acids and phytonutrients.

I recommend one scoop one to two times a day mixed with the fiber supplement. I find it best to take this upon awakening. Do not take Green Superfood in the evening since it is very stimulating and may cause insomnia. However, all the ingredients are natural and contain no stimulants such as caffeine or ephedra.

I personally start my morning as soon as I awaken with two scoops of Ultrafiber, one scoop of Green Superfood, one-half fresh, squeezed lemon or lime and 8 ounces of water. I place this in a shaker cup, shake it for about twenty seconds and then drink. Stevia can be added to sweeten it.

High-chloropyll foods not only boost the immune system, but they also help to improve both digestion and elimination.

Candida Medications

In addition to supplements and herbs, I commonly use medications to control candida.

Nystatin

Nystatin is an antifungal antibiotic that is able to kill a wide variety of different types of yeast. Most folks can take it without side effects. Nystatin tends to stay in the GI tract and do its work instead of being absorbed into other parts of the body. Nystatin is even safe for infants to use. But because Nystatin is poorly absorbed, it may not be as effective for candida that has attacked the entire body.

Ask your doctor about prescribing this medication for you.

A Candida-Busting Cocktail

For a very mild case of candida, I simply recommend 1000 milligrams of caprylic acid three times a day with meals and 500 milligrams of garlic three times a day.

Here's what I prescribe to those experiencing a mild to moderate case of candida:

- Nystatin, 1,000,000 units three times a day
- Caprylic acid, 1000 mg. three times a day
- Garlic, 500 mg. three times a day

If the yeast problem does not go away, I may add any of the following:

- Grapefruit seed extract, 200 mg. three times a day
- Oil of oregano, three 50-mg. tablets three times a day
- Tanalbit, three capsules three times a day
- Goldenseal, 500 mg. three times a day

If the infection is very severe I will often use the medication Diflucan.

Diflucan

Diflucan is so powerful that a single 150-milligram tablet can treat a vaginal candida infection. If your candida overgrowth is severe, you may need to take Diflucan anywhere from a few weeks up to as long as a month.

There are many other medications for yeast

available. However, I believe that these are the safest ones presently available.

Detoxing for Dynamic Results

When candida herbs or medications are taken, yeast die-off reactions commonly occur. This die-off reaction is called a "Herxheimer Reaction." When your body begins rapidly killing off the candida, it may absorb large amounts of the yeast cell particles and toxins.

If you are experiencing this reaction, these symptoms may occur: gas, headaches, fatigue, muscle aches,

> *Restore us, O Lord, and bring us back to you again! Give us back the joys we once had!*
> —Lamentations 5:21

joint aches, sinus congestion, sore throat, rashes, dizziness and even depression. These symptoms seldom last longer than a few days or up to a week after starting yeast herbs or medications.

The answer to this sloughing off of dead yeast is detoxing. As your body goes through this process, detoxing will help your body cleanse itself from this increase of toxins.

Liver Detoxification

Not only does candida overgrowth affect the

immune system and GI tract, but it also has a very profound impact upon the liver as well.

Liver detoxification is occurring continually in the body. However, many times the body's detoxification pathways are overwhelmed by yeast, toxins produced by yeast, leaky gut, food allergies and so on. Therefore, herbs and supplements are critically important for supporting and improving liver detoxification.

Liver detoxification takes place in two phases.

Phase 1

During Phase 1 detoxification, destructive toxins are burned or oxidized, which causes them to become more soluble in water. Let me explain. The liver is like a large filter and is designed to remove toxic material such as drugs, chemicals, dead cells, toxins, yeast bacteria and other microorganisms. The liver has two main detoxification pathways for breaking down and removing these toxic substances. The pathways are called Phase 1 and Phase 2 detoxification. Phase 1 converts a toxin to a less harmful toxin. This is done through chemical reactions, which can in turn produce large amounts of free radicals that can further damage the liver cells.

This process tends to produce free radicals.

Free radicals can also damage liver cells, and they can damage the lining of the intestines as the free radicals are excreted through the bile and then dumped into the GI tract. This in turn can aggravate leaky gut.

Antioxidants never work alone. They work together to help to recycle one another. So I recommend taking a comprehensive antioxidant formula that con-

> *Do not rejoice over me, O my enemy. Though I fall I will rise; though I dwell in darkness, the LORD is a light for me.*
> —MICAH 7:8, NAS

tains plenty of vitamin E, vitamin C, lipoic acid, coenzyme Q_{10}, grape seed and pine bark extract, beta carotene and the minerals copper, zinc, manganese, selenium and sulfur. These can be obtained in Divine Health Multivitamins and Divine Health Antioxidants.

Phase 2

The other phase of liver detoxification is Phase 2 detoxification. In this phase, the chemicals that are oxidized during Phase 1 are joined to an amino acid or another compound to render it less harmful. As the toxin is joined to the amino acid, it becomes water soluble so that it can be excreted from the body by the bile or in the urine.

The most important amino acids for Phase 2 detoxification are cysteine, taurine and methionine, which are sulfur-containing amino acids. Eggs, garlic, onions, cruciferous veggies (cabbage, broccoli, cauliflower, Brussels sprouts), fish, poultry and meats are good sources of sulfur, which aids in Phase 2 detoxification. Choose free-range meat and chicken. At lease one sulfur-containing food should be eaten daily. Cysteine and methionine are also converted into glutathione, which is a potent detoxifier of the liver. It is also an antioxidant.

To assist your body in Phase 2 detoxification, I recommend the following:

- Take N-acetyl cysteine, otherwise known as NAC, and taurine. These supplements will help replenish glutathione stores, which protect the liver from damage from drugs and other toxins. I recommend 500 milligrams of NAC and 500 milligrams of taurine daily.

- Eat at least one serving a week of cruciferous vegetables such as broccoli, cauliflower, Brussels sprouts and cabbage to help to improve liver detoxification.

Restoring Life to Your Liver

Several other supplements will restore your liver to health and vitality.

Milk thistle

Milk thistle contains a bioflavonoid called silymarin that also protects the liver against toxins. Silymarin—the active ingredient in milk thistle—prevents the depletion of glutathione. I recommend 100–200 milligrams of silymarin three times a day.

Glutathione

Glutathione is the most important antioxidant that enables the liver to detoxify. Silymarin can increase the level of glutathione in the liver up to 35 percent. The combination of milk thistle (silymarin) and N-acetyl cysteine (NAC) is extremely important in restoring glutathione levels and thus in protecting and restoring normal liver function. As above, I recommend 100–200 milligrams of silymarin (milk thistle) three times a day and 500 milligrams of NAC once a day.

Lipoic acid

Lipoic acid is also important in increasing the levels of glutathione. I recommend 100–200 milligrams of lipoic acid three times a day for severe candidiasis, and 50–100 milligrams three times a day for moderate candida.

If you have mild candida, all you usually need is a multivitamin and antioxidant formula. If you have severe candidiasis, you will need the multivitamin and antioxidants in addition to supplements of milk thistle, NAC, taurine and extra lipoic acid.

Restoring Friendly Bacteria

When we think of bacteria, most of us think of something negative, such as a bacterial infection. But as we saw earlier, bacteria are not all bad. As a matter of fact, much of the bacteria are very good and vitally important to the proper functioning of our bodies.

On any given day, at least four hundred different varieties of bacteria live and breed in your gastrointestinal tract. That means that approximately a hundred trillion individual bacteria are making residence in your GI tract.

> *Be strong and courageous! Do not be afraid of them! The LORD your God will go ahead of you. He will neither fail you nor forsake you.*
> —DEUTERONOMY 31:6

These are the good guys. They form two different types:

- Lactobacillus acidophilus
- Bifido bacteria

These friendly bacteria live in your small and large intestines all the time, controlling mucus, debris, yeast, parasites and overgrowth of pathogenic (bad) bacteria. They also produce vitamin K and B vitamins, and they maintain the proper pH for the digestive tract.

However, if this healthy population of good bacteria is destroyed or reduced in number, your immune system and liver are forced to work much harder to deal with all the impurities and microorganisms that enter into the blood.

Friendly bacteria also neutralize toxins and cancer-causing chemicals and prevent their absorption back into the bloodstream. Good bacteria produce lactic acid, which inhibits the growth of harmful bacteria such as salmonella, shigella and E. coli. These good bacteria also produce fatty acids that make it difficult for candida to survive.

If your body gets overloaded with harmful bacteria you will suffer many different symptoms.

Bad bacteria cause foul-smelling stools and painful gas, bloating and abdominal cramps, constipation and diarrhea. Good bacteria, on the other hand, stop bad bacteria from growing and relieve painful gas, constipation and diarrhea.

Good bacteria coat the lining of the intestines, forming a protective barrier against invasions by yeast and other microorganisms.

Lactobacillus acidophilus

Lactobacillus acidophilus is powerful against the growth of candida. This good form of bacteria lives in your small intestines all the time. Lactobacillus bifidus lives mainly in your large intestines.

You can be sure that your body has enough of these important bacteria by drinking lactose-free kefir or by eating lactose-, fruit- and sugar-free yogurt as previously mentioned. During a severe attack of candida overgrowth, you can also choose to supplement with good bacteria.

The DDS-1 strain of lactobacillus acidophilus is a super-efficient strain of acidophilus, which is superior in its ability to attach to the lining of the small intestines and help control yeast overgrowth. DDS-1 is a supplement that can be found in most health food stores. It is important to keep it refrigerated. Take 1 teaspoon two to three times a day.

FOS

FOS (otherwise known as fructooligo-saccharides) is a special polysaccharide that is not digested by man, yet feeds friendly bacteria and helps them to grow, while at the same time reducing bad bacteria.

Take 2000 milligrams of FOS a day in order to nourish the good bacteria. You can find FOS at any health food store. It is commonly combined with the acidophilus and bifidus supplements.

You should take at least three to five billion organisms of acidophilus and bifidus bacteria on a daily basis in order to recolonize the GI tract.

> *"For I will restore you to health and I will heal you of your wounds,"* declares the LORD.
> —JEREMIAH 30:17, NAS

This will enable your body to overcome yeast. This is approximately 1 teaspoon of acidophilus/bifidus two times a day. This should also contain FOS. I recommend BioDophilus-FOS from Biotics, which contains DDS-1 acidophilus, bifidus bacteria and FOS in the recommended dosage.

Healing Your Gut

Candida overgrowth is war that takes place in your gut. Yeast may damage and may even partially destroy the lining of the gastrointestinal tract. That's why it is very important to help your body to heal this war zone.

To heal the lining of the GI tract, I recommend the following supplements:

- L-glutamine, ½–1 tsp. three times a day
- N-acetyl-glucosamine, 500 mg. three times a day
- Gamma oryzanol, which is found in rice bran, 300 mg. daily
- FOS, 200 mg. daily
- Colostrum, one to two 500-mg. capsules three times a day

These supplements can be purchased from a health food store or from a nutritionist.

Two products that I use contain most of these supplements. They are IPS from Biotics and Total Leaky Gut from Nutri-West. I recommend one to two tablets of each three times a day thirty minutes before meals. These are commonly recommended by nutritionists and nutritional doctors.

Supplements to Strengthen Immunity

Your body's immune system is your first line of

defense against the ravages of a yeast attack. Therefore, it's vitally important to strengthen your immune system as much as possible. Here are some important vitamins that will arm your body to wage war against yeast overgrowth.

Sending your immune system to battle against candida overgrowth without giving it vital nutrients and minerals is like sending an army to war without guns. If your body is lacking B_5, B_6, B_{12}, folic acid, vitamin C, vitamin E, vitamin A, selenium, zinc and essential fatty acids, as well as protein, you could be in trouble. It's important to supply your body with the equipment it needs.

Lack of sleep also impairs immune function. Medications such as corticosteroids and antibiotics may deplete the body of B vitamins and zinc, thus impairing immune function. Alcohol and cigarette smoke also impair the immune system.

To be sure that your immune system has the equipment it needs to do its job, here are some important supplements you need to battle candidiasis.

A good multivitamin/multimineral supplement

A deficiency of certain nutrients is probably

the most common cause for a poorly functioning immune system. Most Americans are deficient in at least one nutrient. Since a deficiency in any nutrient can result in decreased function of the immune system, it is critically important to take a comprehensive multivitamin and mineral supplement on a daily basis. I recommend Divine Health Multivitamins.

The thymus is a major player in the functioning of your immune system. It orchestrates the working of your immune system throughout your life. When you are born, this gland is larger than your heart. But as you age it gets increasingly smaller. This reduction in size directly corresponds to your immune system's ability to produce disease-fighting T-cells.

Several nutrients can actually prevent this thymus shrinkage. They include:

- Vitamin C
- Vitamin E
- Beta carotene
- Selenium
- Zinc

Vitamin B_6, zinc and vitamin C are needed to improve thymic hormone function.

You can find these nutrients in a comprehensive multivitamin and mineral supplement such as Divine Health Multivitamins.

Zinc

The most important of these supplements for improving thymus function is zinc. When your thymus lacks zinc, vital T-cells are decreased. Take 20–30 milligrams of zinc per day.

Vitamin C

Taking extra doses of vitamin C is extremely important for improving immune function since T-cells contain high levels of vitamin C. Additionally, everyday stress robs your bodies of vitamin C. Therefore, supplementing vitamin C daily is vital for improving your immune system.

I recommend taking high doses of vitamin C daily, approximately 500–1000 milligrams three times a day. However, it is best to take a buffered form of vitamin C.

Conclusion

The impact of candida is complicated. It ravages vital organs and robs your body of strength and health until it leaves you feeling completely depleted. But thank goodness that is not the end.

With the help of this balanced, well-tested regimen of vitamins, minerals, antioxidants, herbs and other supplements, total restoration for your body is not far away.

But never forget, a doctor can give you a prescription or bind a wound, but only the Great Physician can heal you. Christ is the healer. And regardless of whether you receive a supernatural touch from God or a natural system of vitamins and healthy advice, all healing ultimately comes from Him.

> *But as for me, I will watch expectantly for the LORD; I will wait for the God of my salvation.*
> —MICAH 7:7, NAS

A BIBLE CURE PRAYER
FOR YOU

Dear Lord, thank You for providing natural supplements to help restore my body to the perfect balance You planned for it. Thank You for strengthening my body and renewing it from the ravages of candida. Most of all, I thank You for being my healer. Release Your power into my body to free it from the power of sickness and disease. Restore my health and my strength so that I can serve You better. Amen.

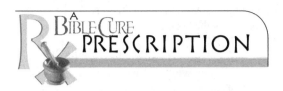

R A BIBLE CURE PRESCRIPTION

Circle the supplements for candida you are planning to take.

Garlic	Goldenseal
Grapefruit extract	Caprylic acid
Oil of oregano	Tanalbit
Chlorophyll supplements	

Circle the medications you plan to discuss with your doctor.

Nystatin   Diflucan

What measures do you plan to take to help your body eliminate dead yeast cell particles and toxins? (circle)

Fiber supplements   Plenty of water

How do you plan to help your body restore good bacteria? (Check the boxes.)

❑ Drink sugar-free and lactose-free kefir, 6–8 ounces a day on an empty stomach

❑ Eat yogurt that does not contain sugar, lactose or fruit, 6–8 ounces a day

❑ Take FOS, DDS-1 acidophilus and bifidus bacteria

What supplements will you take to strengthen immunity? (Check the boxes.)

❑ A comprehensive multivitamin/multi-mineral such as Divine Health Multi-vitamin

❑ A comprehensive antioxidant such as Divine Health Antioxidants

❑ Chlorophyll drink such as Divine Health Green Superfood

What supplements will you take to restore your liver? (circle)

Milk thistle
NAC (N-acetyl cysteine)
Taurine
Lipoic acid

Chapter 4

Recover Your Edge With Lifestyle Changes

A long time ago a king named David experienced a defeat. He and all his people were robbed. Their goods were taken, their wives and children were taken hostage and their city was burned with fire. When David arrived at the scene and realized what his enemies had done, he responded by praying. He asked God, "'Should I chase them? Will I catch them?' And the LORD told him, 'Yes, go after them. You will surely recover everything that was taken from you!'" (1 Sam. 30:8).

In a different kind of way, you may be feeling just as David felt when he came back to his city. Perhaps candida has robbed you of your strength, stolen your health and devastated your body. If so, I suggest you do as David did. Go to God and ask Him for help. As with David, He will help you to recover all that your enemy has robbed from you.

You know, there were times in the Bible when the Israelites didn't have to fight their enemies. God did it for them and they just watched. But other times they had to

> *Is there no medicine in Gilead? Is there no physician there? Why is there no healing for the wounds of my people?*
> —Jeremiah 8:22

go out and fight the battle with God's help. They never regarded one victory as being more from God than the other. They believed God's help was with them in each situation.

Healing is just like that. Sometimes God simply touches a body supernaturally and a person is healed. I've witnessed many such moments of divine intervention. Still, there are other times when God tells us to go and fight our physical battle. But whether we are healed in a sparkling supernatural moment or we go into battle, God's promise is with us as it was with David. He says, "Go, for you will recover all."

This Bible Cure booklet is providing you with weapons for your battle, powerful keys that with God's help will ensure your success. So let's look at another key: lifestyle changes that can give you an edge in your battle.

Do You Get Enough Rest?

Your immune system is dependent upon the rest you give it. If you burn your candle at both ends, eventually the ends will meet at the middle and your immune system will become depleted.

To strengthen your immune system so that it can effectively battle candida, you must sleep at least eight hours at night. Getting enough rest is important all the time, but it's especially important during the battle you're in.

Minimizing Stress

Stress drains your immune system as little else does. Therefore, support your body's fight against yeast by minimizing as much stress in your life as possible.

Here are some pointers:

- Don't work extra hours while your body is battling yeast.
- Don't take on any new projects or new obligations.
- Simplify your life as much as possible until you are well. Learn how to rest, conserve, preserve and rebuild your immune system.

Mercury, a Hidden Enemy

One thing you may not have thought of in your battle against candida is your teeth. If your mouth is full of old amalgam fillings, you may have a hidden enemy.

Your immune system could be suppressed by mercury toxicity, which is usually due to amalgam fillings in the teeth. These are actually silver fillings. Silver fillings are primarily composed of silver, mercury and tin. The mercury contained in these silver fillings is very dangerous to the human body.

If you have silver fillings, then you probably have an overgrowth of candida in your GI tract. Hundreds of published scientific papers directly link the mercury released from these amalgam fillings to chronic disease.

If you have these fillings, mercury is continually being released in your mouth. Every time you brush your teeth, chew gum or drink hot beverages, mercury vapor is released, increasing the release of mercury. In fact, those with amalgam fillings or silver fillings have an average mercury vapor content that's ten times higher than those without silver fillings. About 80 percent of this inhaled mercury vapor is then actually absorbed into your bloodstream.

The mercury that is released in your body binds to the mineral receptor sites for zinc, selenium and other minerals, thus further depressing your immune system.

To speak with a well-informed nutritional doctor who knows how to diagnose and treat mercury toxicity, call 1-800-LEADOUT to find a doctor near you. To find a biological dentist, call GLCCM at (800) 286-6013. If your dentist is not trained in the proper removal of mercury, please call GLCCM and find one who is. Improper removal of silver fillings can seriously impair the immune system, impeding your recovery from candida.

Conclusion

If you have discovered that enemies of toxins and stress have attacked you body even more than you realized, don't be alarmed. Do what David did— look to God for help. God promises never to fail you nor forsake you. The Bible says, "Be strong and courageous, do not be afraid or tremble at them, for the LORD your God is the one who goes with you. He will not fail you or forsake you" (Deut. 31:6, NAS).

With God's help, you will recover all!

A BIBLE CURE PRAYER
FOR YOU

*Dear God, thank You that You promise
total recovery of health and strength to
my body. Thank You that You promise to
never fail me or leave me no matter what
I am battling or going through. Your love
and care for my life mean so much to me.
I am truly grateful. Help me to make the
lifestyle changes necessary to battle my
enemies of sickness and disease, and
most of all, help me to use my good health
and vitality to serve You. Amen.*

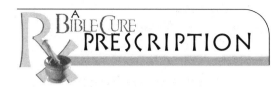

A BIBLE CURE PRESCRIPTION

Write a prayer thanking God for His help in recovering all.

_____

_____

_____

_____

_____

_____

List the things in your life that you want God to help you recover.

_____

_____

_____

_____

_____

_____

Chapter 5

Recharge Your Spirit With Faith

Until now we've looked at many natural things you can do to recover the good health that God intended for you. Let's take a moment to look at the energizing power of faith.

Faith recharges your spirit, giving you the power to reach beyond this material world and take hold of the healing power of God. Hear what the Bible says about faith: "And this is the victory that overcomes the world—our faith" (1 John 5:4, NKJV).

The final key in your Bible cure is the power of faith. This transcendent force has overcome kingdoms and risen above every obstacle.

Depression and stress are perhaps two of the worst things that can happen to your immune system. Both of them can do amazing damage to your body and tremendously impair its ability to function. When you are depressed, your immune system tends to be depressed as well. When you are stressed out, your immune system is stressed, too.

The amount of immune suppression is usually related to the amount of stress you are under. During periods of stress people are far more prone to infection because of the lowered immune function caused by stress.

Take Five

The energizing power of faith will form a mighty shield against the destructive power of stress and depression. Here are five ways to arm yourself.

Take time to relax.

Your body will enter into a deep state of relaxation when you praise and worship God and meditate on the Word of God. Deep-breathing exercises, massages and even taking a hot bath while playing soothing worship music will also greatly relax your body. Praise and worship music gets into your spirit, and the peace it gives provides an internal shield against stress, depression and anxiety.

Get to know your body. Take note of when you feel particularly stressed out and what changes take place. After a particularly stressful day or event, give special attention to relaxing your body and your nerves. A few moments of relaxation will allow your immune system to recover from the damaging effects of stress.

Take a moment to laugh.

Most people battling candida overgrowth are stressed out and depressed. Therefore, they usually have a very low-functioning immune system. Their cortisol and adrenaline levels are usually either elevated or extremely depressed. The best medicine for overcoming stress and depression is laughter. In fact, the Bible says that a merry heart does good like a medicine. (See Proverbs 17:22.)

Norman Cousins wrote the book *Anatomy of an Illness As Perceived by the Patient* in 1979.[1] Cousins used laughter to fight a serious disease, actually laughing his way back to health. He watched funny movies such as the Marx Brothers films. He watched funny TV shows such as *Candid Camera* and read funny books.

A good belly laugh is able to stimulate all the major organs like a massage. Laughter also helps to raise your energy level and helps to pull you out of the pit of depression. Take at least a ten- to twenty- minute laughter break a day. Watch funny movies and TV shows. Read jokes in the newspaper, books or magazines, and share these clean jokes with others because laughter is contagious. Instead of looking critically at a situation, find out what's funny about it.

Joy gives you strength. The Bible says, "Don't be dejected and sad, for the joy of the LORD is your strength!" (Neh. 8:10).

You may be thinking, *That's easy for him to say. He doesn't know my circumstances!* No one but God truly

> *Restore to me again the joy of your salvation, and make me willing to obey you.*
> —PSALM 51:12

knows another's circumstances, thoughts and feelings. But that doesn't matter; you can find joy, not in circumstances, but in Christ. The Bible promises, "Thou wilt make known to me the path of life; in Thy presence is fulness of joy; in Thy right hand there are pleasures forever" (Ps. 16:11, NAS).

I encourage you to find joy in life by knowing Christ.

The average man and woman laughs about four to eight times a day. The average child laughs about 150 times a day. Strengthen your immune system by beginning to laugh more today.

Take refuge in the Scriptures.

God's Word breaks the destructive power of certain deadly emotions such as fear, rage, hatred, resentment, bitterness, shame and so forth. I encourage you to quote scriptures related to them at least three times a day on a continuous basis. Also consider reading and meditating on Bible passages like 1 Corinthians 13, the chapter on love, since there is no greater force in the universe than the power of God's love. It is able to break the bondage of any destructive emotion.

Take up positive attitudes.

Related to Scripture reading is the practice of "putting on" the positive, healthy emotions that it speaks of—emotions like love, joy, peace, patience, kindness, goodness and self-control. We know that certain emotions are associated with lowered immune function and higher cortisol levels. Approaching life with the biblical "attitude prescription" will help you avoid the damaging effects of stress, fear and worry.

A Bible Cure Prayer
FOR YOU

Dear Jesus Christ, thank You for dying on the cross to pay the cost of mankind's sins, including my own. I give You all my sins and repent for each and every one. I ask You to come into my heart and life. And I surrender myself and my future to Your will and to Your care. Thank You for suffering under the Roman lash so that I can be healed and made completely whole. I receive You right now. In Jesus' name, amen.

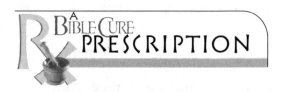

Faith Builder

He was pierced through for our transgressions, He was crushed for our
iniquities; the chastening of our well-
being fell upon Him, and by His scourging we are healed.

—ISAIAH 53:5, NAS

Read this dynamic scripture several times
aloud. It has great power! Insert your own name
into it.

He was pierced through for _____
transgressions, He was crushed for
_____ iniquities; the chastening of
_____ well-being fell upon Him, and
by His scourging _____ is healed!

A PERSONAL NOTE

From Don and Mary Colbert

God desires to heal you of disease. His Word is full of promises that confirm His love for you and His desire to give you His abundant life. His desire includes more than physical health for you; He wants to make you whole in your mind and spirit as well through a personal relationship with His Son, Jesus Christ.

If you haven't met my best friend, Jesus, I would like to take this opportunity to introduce Him to you. It is very simple.

If you are ready to let Him come into your heart and become your best friend, just bow your head and sincerely pray this prayer from your heart:

Lord Jesus, I want to know You as my Savior and Lord. I believe You are the Son of God and that You died for my sins. I also believe You were raised from the dead and now sit at the right hand of the Father praying for me. I ask You to forgive me for my sins and change my heart so that I can

be Your child and live with You eternally.
Thank You for Your peace. Help me to
walk with You so that I can begin to know
You as my best friend and my Lord. Amen.

If you have prayed this prayer, we rejoice with you in your decision and your new relationship with Jesus. Please contact us at pray4me@strang.com so that we can send you some materials that will help you become established in your relationship with the Lord. You have just made the most important decision of your life. We look forward to hearing from you.

Notes

CHAPTER 1:
GET INFORMED

1. Michael Colgan, *The New Nutrition* (San Diego: C. I. Publications, 1994).
2. William G. Crook, *The Yeast Connection Handbook* (Jackson, TN: Professional Books, 1999), 15–19.
3. Adapted from Crook, *The Yeast Connection Handbook*, 15–19.

CHAPTER 2:
RESTORE YOUR HEALTH WITH NUTRITION

1. For more information on the glycemic index, see the glycemic index chart in *The Bible Cure for Weight Loss and Muscle Gain*, 12–15.

CHAPTER 5:
RECHARGE YOUR SPIRIT WITH FAITH

1. Norman Cousins, *Anatomy of an Illness As Perceived by the Patient* (Norton, NY: Bantam, 1979).
2. S. I. McMillen, *None of These Diseases* (Westwood, NJ: Revell, 1963), 7.

Don Colbert, M.D., was born in Tupelo, Mississippi. He attended Oral Roberts School of Medicine in Tulsa, Oklahoma, where he received a bachelor of science degree in biology in addition to his degree in medicine. Dr. Colbert completed his internship and residency with Florida Hospital in Orlando, Florida. He is board certified in family practice and has received extensive training in nutritional medicine.

If you would like more information about natural and divine healing, or information about ***Divine Health Nutritional Products***®, you may contact Dr. Colbert at:

DR. DON COLBERT

1908 Boothe Circle
Longwood, FL 32750
Telephone: 407-331-7007
(For ordering products only)

Dr. Colbert's website is www.drcolbert.com.

Disclaimer: Dr. Colbert and the staff of Divine Health Wellness Center are prohibited from addressing a patient's medical condition by phone, facsimile or e-mail. Please refer questions related to your medical condition to your own primary care physician.

Announcing

Powerful new Divine Health products to help you live in the wonderful joy of God's divine health for you!

Divine Health™ Candida Formula

A powerful combination of anti-yeast agents and herbs beneficial to the liver and gastrointestinal tract make up our Candida Formula. Our formula contains pau d'arco, grapefruit seed extract, biotin, sodium caprylate, oregano leaf extract, berberine sulfate, cinnamon bark extract, goldenseal root extract and much more. You don't have to suffer from symptoms of yeast overgrowth; the ingredients in this product will help you keep the yeast syndrome in check, while you build your immune system. Improve your health with this natural candida remedy.